HeartyNFit

FISAYO ADEGOKE, DHSC

Paperback ISBN: 978-1-965593-44-8

Printed in the United States of America.

DISCLAIMER

The information provided in this journal is for general knowledge and informational purpose. Always consult with your healthcare provider for any health concerns and decisions related to your health or treatment.

The meal guides are a general guide for those who want to start eating healthy and do not have any underlying conditions such as diabetes, etc. If you are on any medication, do not skip your medications or stop without your doctor's supervision. Information provided in this journal is not intended to be a substitute for professional medical advice, diagnosis or treatment.

For Health Coaching and Wellness Consultation: 202-643-4648 or drfisayoadegoke@gmail.com

INTRODUCTION

A few years ago, I went for my annual physical examination, and I was asked to do the lipid profile test. The results indicated that my cholesterol (LDL) was high. As a nutrition student, I understood the meaning of the results and what it meant if the cholesterol levels were high. The doctor told me that I needed a lifestyle change to improve my eating habits and be back in 6 months or a year. He said if nothing changes by then, I will have to start taking medications. Right there in the place, I was determined to improve my eating habits and get a change in my cholesterol levels. I told my doctor I would love to have my cholesterol levels checked in six months. I left the annual visit thinking about how I could help myself. I became intentional about my eating habits and exercise routines. My cholesterol levels improved when I went for a follow-up visit. In this heart health guide, I will be sharing some helpful information that can help you improve your blood cholesterol level, just like mine did!

If you need to lower your blood cholesterol levels or you have high blood pressure, lifestyle modification can help improve your numbers and also reduce your risk of heart disease.

UNDERSTANDING HEART DISEASE

Did you know the heart is a muscular organ that beats 115,000 times a day? It pumps about 2,000 gallons of blood daily and exactly eight pints of blood 24/7. It gives life to your body, and you cannot afford to take your heart health with levity. You don't have to develop hypertension, diabetes, or high blood cholesterol levels before you adjust your lifestyle and if you already have any of these conditions, it is not the end of the world. You can manage the conditions with lifestyle changes coupled with instructions given to you by your doctor.

Heart disease can be described as various types of conditions that affect the heart's structure and function. All heart diseases are cardiovascular diseases, but not all cardiovascular diseases are heart diseases. There are around 620 million people living with heart and circulatory diseases globally, and about 60 million people (about twice the population of Texas and almost the population of the UK) develop a heart or circulatory disease annually. Cardiovascular disease is the leading cause of death worldwide, killing an estimated 17.9 million lives yearly.

Heart disease is the leading cause of death for women in the United States. About 314,186 died of the disease in 2020. One out of five females dies because of disease. One-third of them die due to cardiovascular disease worldwide.

According to the American Heart Association, more than one in three men have heart disease in the United States. The most common type in the United

States is coronary artery disease, which is also known as CAD. It affects the flow of blood to the heart, and when this happens, there is a decrease in blood flow to the heart, and a heart attack occurs.

Coronary heart disease cannot be cured, but treatment can help manage the symptoms, thereby reducing the risk of having problems such as heart attacks. Treatments include lifestyle changes such as having a regular exercise routine, healthy eating and tobacco cessation for those who smoke. Some other heart diseases are high blood pressure and high blood cholesterol levels.

In this eBook, I will be focusing more on high blood cholesterol levels, their causes, and how to improve your cholesterol levels and blood pressure numbers.

The meal and exercise plans are provided as a guide to help with meal ideas and exercise routines on your wellness journey. The healthy habit and blood pressure trackers are provided to help you track your habits and monitor your blood pressure regularly.

WHAT CAUSES HEART DISEASE?

The most common risk factors for heart disease and stroke are high blood pressure, high low-density lipoprotein (LDL) cholesterol, diabetes, smoking and secondhand smoke exposure, obesity, unhealthy diet, and physical inactivity.

SYMPTOMS OF HEART DISEASE

Most of the time, heart disease may be silent and not noticed or diagnosed except when an individual experiences signs such as chest pain or discomfort, dizziness, chest palpitations, shortness of breath, and fatigue.

The signs and symptoms of heart disease include chest pain, dizziness, and shortness of breath. Knowing these signs may help males to reduce their risk of developing severe complications.

Men are more likely to experience heart attack symptoms such as crushing chest pain, squeezing, discomfort in the chest, and pain in the arm, back, or jaw. Other symptoms include shortness of breath, cold sweat, and nausea.

Women are less likely to experience crushing chest pain. However, they experience symptoms such as pain in the jaw, neck, or chest, lightheadedness or feeling faint, squeezing on the upper back, and pressure or squeezing on the upper back instead.

Consequently, women are more likely to ignore their cardiac symptoms as it is less obvious that they relate specifically to the heart.

Almost 50% of premature deaths may be due to unhealthy lifestyle habits. Thereby increasing the risk of developing heart disease or other lifestyle-related diseases, including diabetes and some cancers. You can reduce your risk of developing heart disease by 90% through lifestyle changes.

Both genders may have chest pain as symptoms, but the chest pain in women is often described by women as a pressure or tightness in the chest. It is also possible to have a heart attack without chest pain.

Women can have symptoms when resting; emotional stress can trigger heart attack symptoms in women. Low levels of estrogen can also increase the risk of heart disease in women. However, lifestyle changes can reduce these risks.

Men are more likely to have chest pain, and women have chest discomfort, nausea, extreme fatigue, and shortness of breath.

High blood pressure does not give you signs; most people can have high blood pressure without knowing they have the disease. That is why you should always check your blood pressure. Some people experience headaches slightly or persistently; therefore, if you notice a persistent headache, check your blood pressure and see your physician without delay.

Having a family history of hypertension is a risk factor for developing it, therefore, take control of your heart health.

There is a difference between being healthy and looking good. You can look good and be unhealthy. High blood pressure has no symptoms. As a busy person who is always on the go, check your blood pressure regularly, at least every other day.

Don't eat too much than your body needs. Overeating can cause obesity, a risk factor for heart disease. If you want to improve your heart health improve your blood pressure, and cholesterol numbers, you need to get rid of excess body weight. To lose excess body weight, you must eat less calories and exercise more.

For example, if an individual eats about 3,000 calories a day, cut back on the amount of daily calories, maybe by 500 calories. At the end of that week, this individual had 17,500 calories instead of the usual 21,000 calories. That's 3,500 calories reduction, which is equivalent to 1 lb. Now imagine adding exercise to it daily and consistently over time. This individual will be able to lose weight, keep it off if consistent, and improve his or her heart health.

KNOW YOUR BMI:

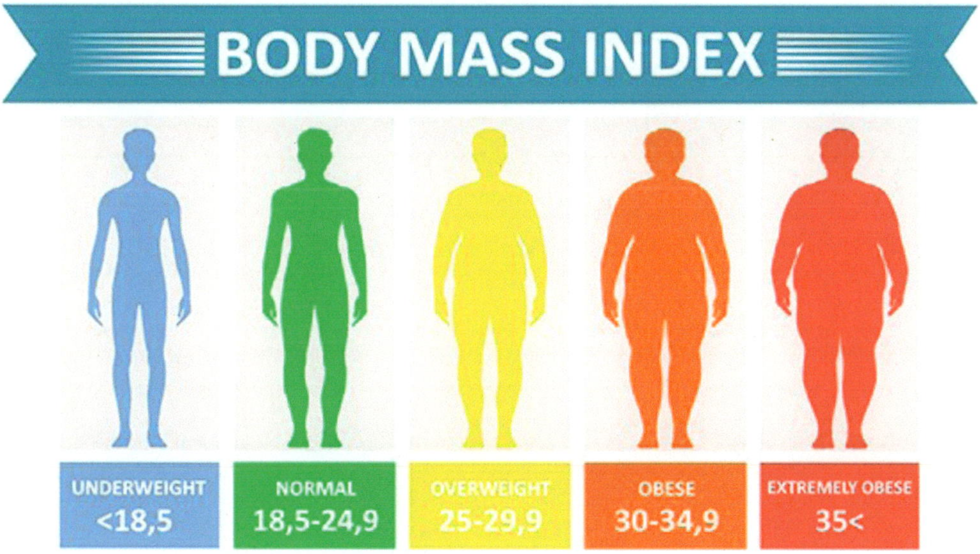

Source: Centers for Disease Control and Prevention (CDC).

Notes Date........... /...........

Notes Date........... /...........

Notes Date........... /...........

Notes Date........... /...........

Notes Date............ /............

Notes Date............ /............

METABOLIC SYNDROME

A Metabolic syndrome is a group of conditions that can increase the risk of heart disease, diabetes, and stroke. It is also called insulin resistance syndrome. Drinking your water regularly may help prevent and treat metabolic syndrome. Water suppresses vasopressin, a hormone linked to fructose-induced obesity, and diabetes.

Someone meets the criteria for metabolic syndrome if:

- Waist circumference is more than 40 in men or 35 in women.
- Triglycerides are 150mg/dL or more.
- Low levels of HDL. Less than 40mg/dL in men, 50mg/dL in women.
- Blood pressure of 130/85 or higher
- High fasting blood sugar of 100mg/dL

If you have any of these, a change of lifestyle is needed.

PLAQUES

Plaques form when cholesterol lodges in the walls of the arteries; this is called atherosclerosis. If blood pressure spikes, probably due to stress, it puts pressure on the plaque's thin wall. This can break open, and a clot is formed. This can lead to a heart attack. Most major heart attacks occur when plaques are ruptured. When plaques don't rupture but enlarge over time, they can block the flow of blood, causing angina (chest pain that may be caused by emotional stress). These blockages are not healthy! They can cause heart attacks or even stroke. That is why you need to be intentional about your eating habits and lifestyle choices.

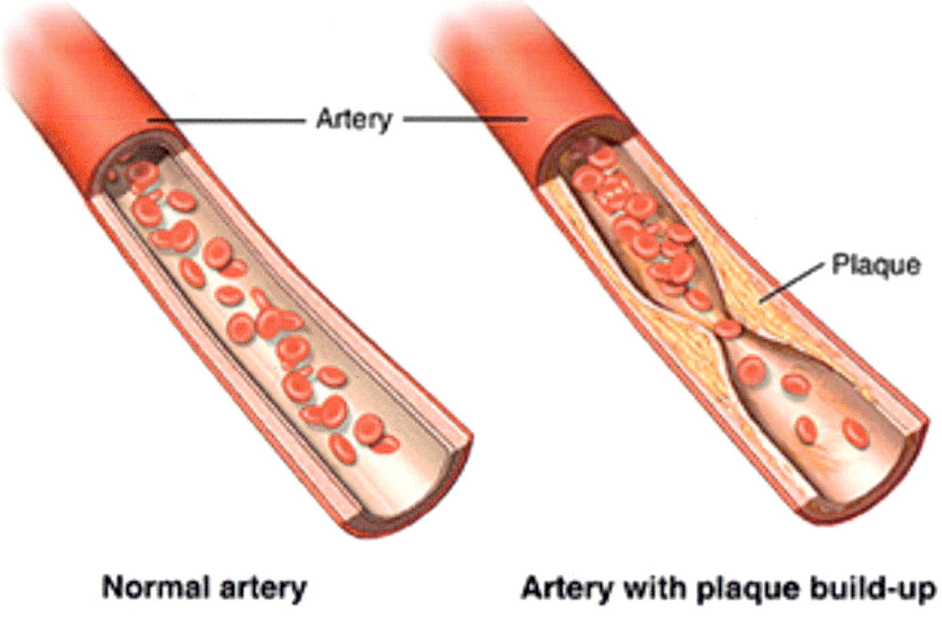

Source: Atherosclerosis Johns Hopkins Medicine.

CHOLESTEROL

Cholesterol is a waxy substance. The body needs it to build cells and make vitamins and other hormones. But too much of it can cause health problems.

There are two sources of cholesterol: the liver, and foods from animals. The liver produces all the cholesterol the body needs, and the remaining cholesterol in the body comes from foods from animals. For example, meat, poultry, and dairy products all contain dietary cholesterol, all of which are high in saturated and trans-fat. These fats cause the liver to make more cholesterol than it otherwise would. Therefore, some people end up having more than needed cholesterol in their bodies. Then, the cholesterol levels go from normal to unhealthy.

UNDERSTANDING YOUR CHOLESTEROL LEVELS.

When the lipid profile test is done, total cholesterol, triglycerides, HDL, and LDL cholesterol are checked and reported.

HDL cholesterol is the "good" cholesterol that reduces the risk of heart disease. It is called "good" cholesterol because it moves cholesterol to the liver so it can be removed from the body. However, a low level of HDL cholesterol increases the risk.

LDL cholesterol is the "bad" cholesterol that causes plaques to build up in the walls of the arteries. High levels of LDL cholesterol increase the risk of heart disease.

High levels of triglycerides can increase the risk of heart disease, especially in women.

RISK FACTORS FOR HIGH CHOLESTEROL.

There are various risk factors for high cholesterol in the blood. Some can be controlled, while some factors cannot be controlled. Controllable factors are diet, exercise, smoking, being overweight, type 2 diabetes, high blood pressure. diet, exercise, smoking, and being overweight, while uncontrollable factors are age, genetics, gender, ethnicity, and family history.

Here are the ranges for total cholesterol in adults; results are given in milligrams per deciliter (mg/dL):

- Normal: Less than 200 mg/dL
- Borderline high: 200 to 239 mg/dL
- High: At or above 240 mg/dL

These are the adult ranges for LDL cholesterol:

- Optimal: Less than 100 mg/dL (This is the goal for people with diabetes or heart disease.)

- Near optimal: 100 to 129 mg/dL
- Borderline high: 130 to 159 mg/dL
- High: 160 to 189 mg/dL
- Very high: 190 mg/dL and higher

The above numbers are general guidelines. The goals will depend on the number of risk factors you have for heart disease.

Your HDL cholesterol levels should be above 40 mg/dL. This type of fat is good for you as it lowers your risk of heart disease. The higher the number, the lower your risk. Sixty mg/dL or above is considered the level to protect you from having heart disease.

High levels of triglycerides are linked with a higher heart disease risk. Here are the adult ranges:

- Normal: Less than 150 mg/dL
- Borderline high: 150 to 199 mg/dL
- High: 200 to 499 mg/dL
- Very high: Above 500 mg/dL

The test results will help your healthcare provider decide if you need lifestyle changes or medications to lower your cholesterol.

Cholesterol Levels

	Total Cholesterol	LDL Cholesterol	HDL Cholesterol
DANGEROUS	**240 and higher**	**160 and higher**	**Under 40** (male) **Under 50** (female)
AT-RISK	**200 – 239**	**100 – 159**	**40-59** (male) **50-59** (female)
HEART-HEALTHY	**Under 200**	**Under 100**	**60 and higher**

Source: clevelandclinic.org

Blood pressure chart: Below is a chart showing blood pressure categories:

BLOOD PRESSURE CATEGORY	SYSTOLIC mm Hg (upper number)		DIASTOLIC mm Hg (lower number)
NORMAL	LESS THAN 120	and	LESS THAN 80
ELEVATED	120 – 129	and	LESS THAN 80
HIGH BLOOD PRESSURE (HYPERTENSION) STAGE 1	130 – 139	or	80 – 89
HIGH BLOOD PRESSURE (HYPERTENSION) STAGE 2	140 OR HIGHER	or	90 OR HIGHER
HYPERTENSIVE CRISIS (consult your doctor immediately)	HIGHER THAN 180	and/or	HIGHER THAN 120

Source: American Heart Association

Notes Date........... /...........

Notes Date........... /...........

Notes Date............ /............

Notes Date............ /............

Notes

Date............ /............

Notes

Date............ /............

DIET AND LIFESTYLE CHANGE

Some diet and lifestyle changes to help improve your blood pressure and blood cholesterol numbers:

There are several lifestyle changes that can help reduce your risk of developing heart disease or having a heart attack.

These include:

- Tobacco cessation
- Maintaining a healthy weight
- Doing at least 150 minutes a week of moderate aerobic exercise or 75 minutes of vigorous aerobic exercise
- Eating a diet low in processed sugars and meat
- Reducing salt consumption
- Increasing the amount of fiber, vegetables, and fruit in the diet
- Having regular checkups to discover any developing health problems earlier.
- Reducing stress through meditation, exercising, and spending time with family and friends.
- Being aware of snoring as a potential sign of heart disease

USING SPICES AND HERBS

Spices and herbs are rich sources of antioxidants. They are used in food and beverages to enhance flavor, aroma and color. They are also used to treat some diseases due to their excellent antioxidant properties.

Examples of spices are:

- Turmeric.
- Ginger.
- Cumin.
- Peppermint.
- Echinacea.
- Cinnamon.
- Chili powder.
- Parsley.

Apart from their antioxidant properties, they are anti-inflammatory, and some spices help improve cognitive functioning.

When cooking, add some spices first and let it cook for a while so the flavors go into the food before adding salt. This will prevent the food from being too salty because these spices have some sodium content in them.

Notes Date............ /............

Notes Date............ /............

Notes Date............ /............

Notes Date............ /............

Notes Date............ /............

Notes Date............ /............

EATING FRUITS AND VEGETABLES

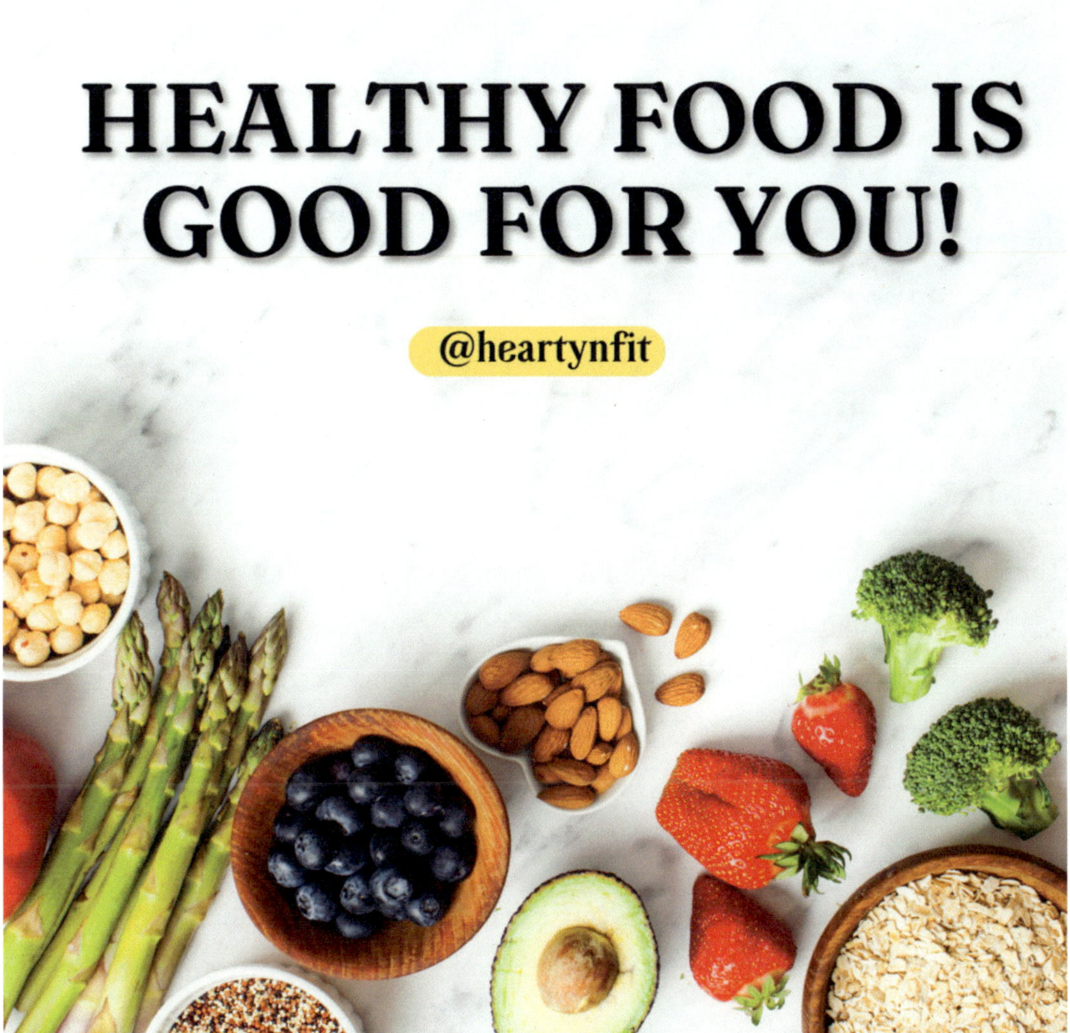

Depending on age and sex, federal guidelines recommend that adults should eat at least one-half to two cups per day of fruit and two to three cups per day of vegetables. Not all people eat the recommended amount of fruits and vegetables every day; this puts them at risk for chronic diseases like diabetes and heart disease. Dietary guidelines recommend five servings of fruits and vegetables every day, including if or not you have diabetes. Since fruits have more calories and sugar than vegetables, try to strike a balance. You can break up your five servings into three vegetable servings and two fruit servings. When it comes to vegetables, people with diabetes should eat at least three servings a day. Vegetables are healthy, full of vitamins and minerals, and some give you a lot of fiber, which helps in reducing your risks of heart disease and other lifestyle-related diseases.

OMEGA-3 FATTY ACIDS

Omega-3 fatty acids are one of the macronutrients that everyone should consume.

They are a good source of healthy fats that can Help lower blood cholesterol levels, Strengthen blood vessels, Lower plaque buildups, Reduce the risk of diabetes, Some forms of cancers and rheumatoid arthritis, Also decrease overall joint pain.

Good food or healthy food indeed is medicine. Having a healthy diet with omega-3s is good for your heart and overall well-being. Reducing the intake of red meat can help you lower your cholesterol levels. If you really love red meat, choose beef sirloin, lamb chops, or top sirloin steak. In short, the loins, round, and chops. However, goat meat is a healthier alternative to other red meats like beef, lamb, and pork. It is nutritious and naturally lean, and its consumption is very beneficial to health. It has less fat, less saturated fat, more iron, and about the same amount of protein compared to beef, pork, lamb, or chicken. Goat meat may help with weight loss goals, and it supplies iron, potassium, zinc, and vitamin B12.

Honeydew melon is good for heart health. It can help in lowering blood cholesterol, however, don't eat too much if you are diabetic. It can elevate blood sugar levels if overeaten. Apples are also good for lowering cholesterol due to their high fiber content. Berries, avocados, pears, oranges, and lemons are good for you.

STOP OVEREATING.

Mindful eating is about awareness of your physical cues, and feelings about food. Paying closer attention to your food and how it makes you feel. It helps to reduce disordered eating behaviors and supports weight loss. Mindful eating is a strategy that helps you better manage your eating habits. It has been shown to reduce binge eating, promote weight loss, and helps you feel better.

Here are some ways to be present at your meal:

- Eat slowly and without distraction
- listen to physical hunger cues and stop eating when you're full
- Eat to maintain overall health and wellness
- Avoid late-night snacking

To overcome the habit of late-night snacking, make sure you eat well during the day. Have a healthy breakfast, lunch, dinner, and if possible, some healthy snacks in between your meals. This way, you will not be too hungry at night.

Portion control tips that can help you no matter how busy you are:

Meal planning: Take a few minutes each week to plan your meals and snacks. This way, you can pre-portion your meals, pack them in convenient containers, and have them ready to grab and go when you're in a hurry.

Mindful eating: Practice mindful eating whenever it's time to have your meals. Slow down, savor each bite, and listen to your body's hunger and fullness cues. Your first feeling of fullness is an indication that you have had enough; if you have to remove your belt when eating a meal, you have eaten too much! Mindful eating and your body's fullness cues help you eat just the right amount, even when you're busy.

Choose Single Servings: When you're purchasing snacks or treats, opt for single-serving packs instead of buying in bulk. This way, you won't be tempted to eat more than you need, and you'll have built-in portion control.

Mind Your Plate Size: Be mindful of the size of your plates and bowls. Using smaller plates can trick your brain into thinking you're eating more; this helps you feel satisfied with smaller meal portions.

By practicing portion control, even on your busiest days, you can nourish your body while staying on track with your wellness goals.

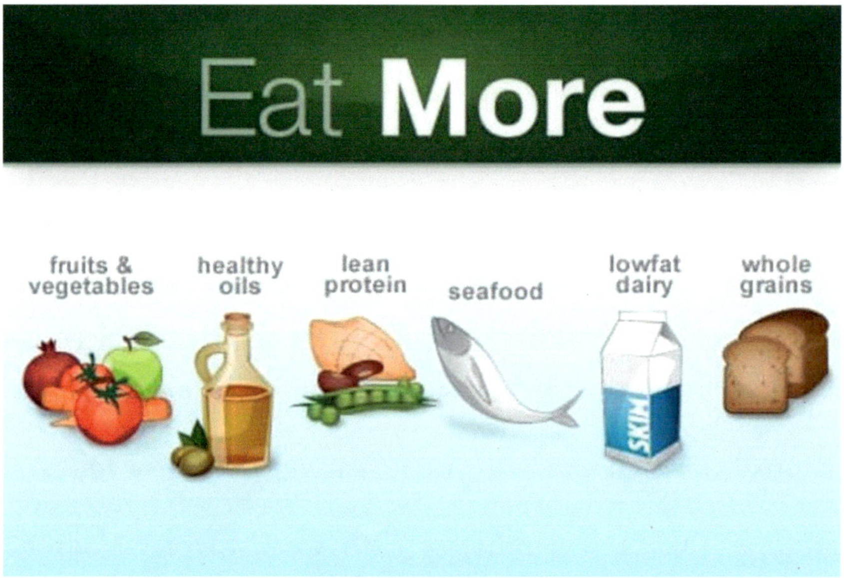

Source: webmd.com

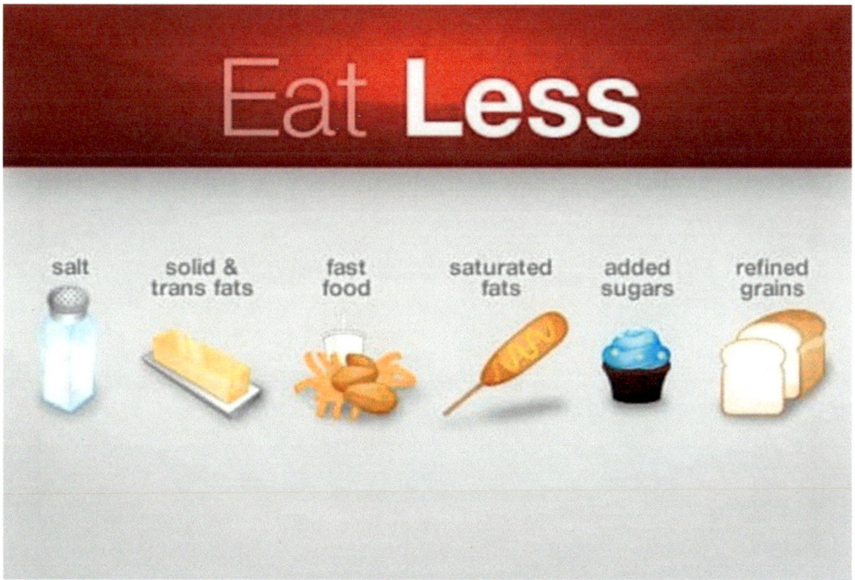

Source: webmd.com

This is a visual reminder of how your plate should be when you eat:

Vegetables should make up the most significant section, followed by grains. Fruits and vegetables fill half the plate, while proteins and grains fill the second half. You can substitute dairy with water if you are allergic to dairy or you do not take dairy.

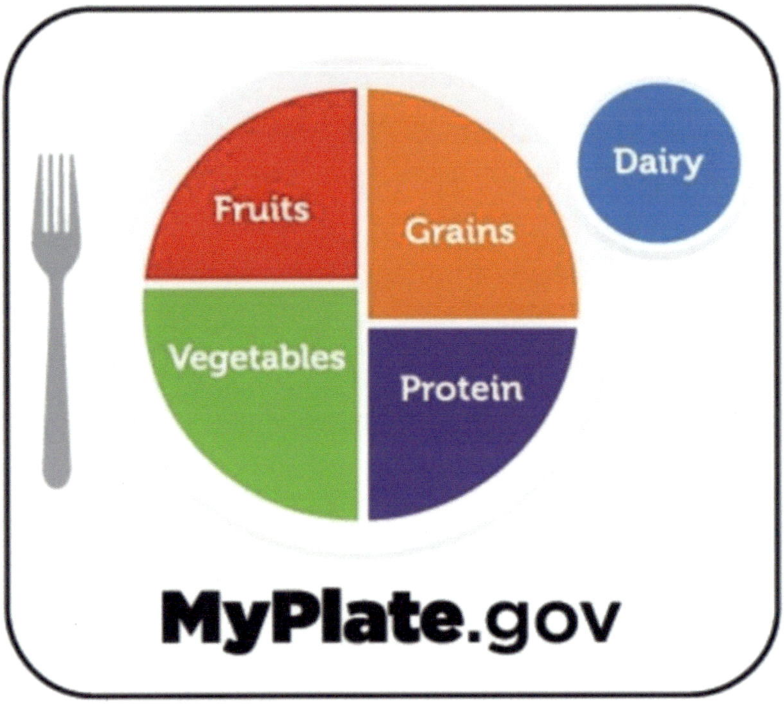

Source: myplate.gov

EXERCISE REGULARLY

If you are busy and don't always have time to exercise. You can start with 5-10 minutes of exercise daily and increase the duration as time goes on. Remember to check with your physician before you do vigorous exercises. Aerobic exercises such as walking, jumping rope, dancing, jogging, swimming, cycling, etc., are good for your heart health. An individual who has hypertension should perform at least 150 minutes per week of moderate-intensity and muscle-strengthening exercise twice a week when there are no specific contraindications.

Regular exercise can bring blood pressure down to safer levels. Some examples of aerobic exercise that can help lower blood pressure include walking, jogging, cycling, swimming, or dancing. At least 30 minutes of daily exercise can help improve blood pressure and cholesterol levels. Examples of strength training exercises include lifting weights, climbing stairs, [cycling], dancing, and doing push-ups, sit-ups and squats. Remember to check with your physician before you start an exercise regimen to be sure you are fit for it.

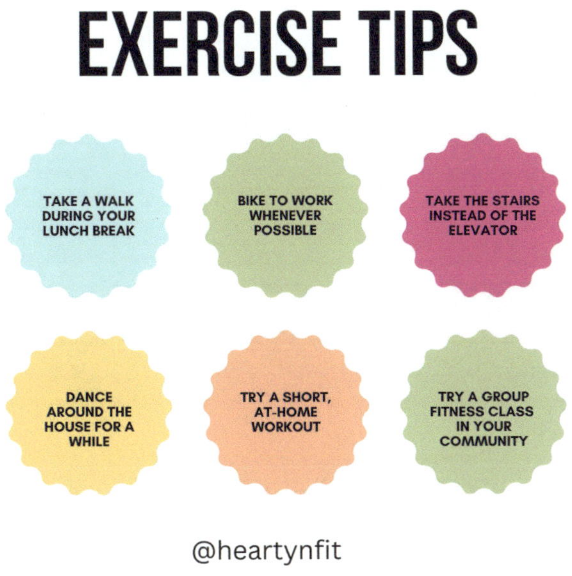

Notes Date............ /............

Notes Date............ /............

Notes Date............/............

....

....

....

....

....

....

....

....

....

....

....

....

Notes Date............/............

....

....

....

....

....

....

....

....

....

....

....

....

Notes Date............ /............

Notes Date............ /............

CHOLESTEROL LOWERING FOODS

FOODS TO IMPROVE CHOLESTEROL LEVELS NATURALLY.

Here are some tips to help you improve your cholesterol level:

- Eat more soluble fiber like oats, oatmeal, and high-fiber foods. It reduces the absorption of cholesterol into your bloodstream.
- Reduce your intake of saturated fats that are found in red meat and full-fat dairy foods.
- Drink more water.
- Regular exercise can help increase the good cholesterol (HDL cholesterol).
- Be intentional about what you put in your body. Your health is your wealth.

WHAT TO EAT

What should you eat? Focus on eating foods low in saturated and trans fats, such as: • A variety of fruits and vegetables. • A variety of whole-grain foods like whole grain bread, cereal, pasta and brown rice. At least half of the servings should be whole grains. • Fat-free, 1% and low-fat milk products. • Poultry without skin and lean meats. When you choose to eat red meat and pork, select options labeled "loin" and "round." These cuts usually have the least amount of fat. • Fatty fish such as salmon, albacore tuna and sardines. Enjoy at least 8 ounces of non-fried fish each week, which may be divided over two servings. • Unsalted nuts, seeds, and legumes (dried beans or peas). • Nontropical vegetable oils like canola, corn, olive or safflower oils.

Other heart-healthy foods include:

- Bitter-leaf soup, also known as ewuro.
- Jute leaves, also known as ewedu.
- Unripe Plantain Flour.
- Avocado.
- Zobo (Hibiscus Drink, unsweetened is best).
- Plantain fufu
- Olive oil is the healthiest when compared to groundnut oil and palm oil
- Fish due to omega-3 fatty acids, which is very good for the heart
- Dark chocolate
- Hausa Koko (Ghanian meal)
- Koose (Ghanian)
- Garden egg stew

Foods to limit:

What should you limit?

- Foods with a lot of sodium (salt).
- Sweets and sugar-sweetened beverages.
- Red meats and fatty meats that aren't trimmed.
- Full-fat dairy products such as whole milk, cream, ice cream, butter, and cheese.
- Baked goods made with saturated and trans fats, like donuts, cakes and cookies.
- Foods that list the words "hydrogenated oils" in the ingredients panel.
- Tropical oils such as coconut, palm and palm kernel oils.
- Solid fats like shortening, stick margarine and lard.
- Fried foods

Notes Date........... /...........

Notes Date........... /...........

Notes Date............ /............

Notes Date............ /............

Notes Date........... /...........

Notes Date........... /...........

HEALTHY LIFESTYLE TIPS FOR THE BUSY INDIVIDUAL

Life can get hectic, and it is easy to get caught up in this fast-paced world we live in. However, don't forget the power of real foods. As a busy person, it is important to have enough nutrients to nourish your body by eating real foods. Consume more 'real foods' and limit the intake of processed foods like canned, boxed or convenience foods. Real foods are nutritious, contain minerals, fibers, antioxidants and other nutrients. Not all processed food is bad, but limit their consumption. Purchase lean protein foods such as tofu, plain greek yogurt, egg, chicken breast, beans, lentils, quinoa, tuna, and salmon, choose foods that have fewer calories and added ingredients.

Studies show that an increase in high levels of cortisol because of long-term stress can increase blood cholesterol, triglycerides, blood sugar, and blood pressure. Therefore, if you are undergoing a lot of stress, then you are at risk of high blood cholesterol levels and blood pressure. That is one of the reasons you have elevated blood cholesterol levels and why some people suffer from hypertension. Too much stress can lead to hypertension. Some conditions like obesity and diabetes can increase your risk of hypertension.

Some time ago, I had high blood cholesterol levels due to too much stress and unhealthy eating habits. Even though I understood the importance of healthy eating, I was not taking the right actions regarding it.

There's a plethora of information on healthy eating now, and almost everyone knows that they should have healthy eating habits. However, knowing is not equivalent to taking action. That is why you need to be intentional about your health. Stress can cause short-term spikes in your blood pressure. These brief and sudden spikes can damage blood vessels or cause heart attacks. Therefore, you need to manage stress well. Anxiety, depression, and being lonely can increase your stress levels. When you reduce your stress levels, the short spikes that can sometimes cause heart attacks or strokes are reduced. Note that anxiety, depression, or being lonely doesn't cause hypertension, but episodes can cause temporary spikes in blood pressure.

Some ways to manage **or minimize stress:**

1. Get enough sleep. Having adequate sleep can help reduce stress and help you live a healthy life. Lack of adequate sleep, insomnia, and sleep apnea can increase the risk of hypertension, obesity, type 2 diabetes, and heart disease. Use these tips to get a better night's sleep:
2. Do some stress-relieving exercises such as walking, dancing, listening to music, gardening, taking a bath, swimming etc.
3. Remove electronic devices and phones away from your bed. Stop the use of electronic devices at least 1 hour before bedtime.
4. Try to go to bed and wake up at the same time each day.
5. Adjust your schedules; do not bite more than you can chew. If you need to delegate or outsource, please do.
6. Take slow, deep breaths; this will help you relax.
7. Exercising regularly can help reduce stress (remember to check with your physician before you start exercising if you have not been exercising for a while).

PRIORITIZE SELF-CARE

Self-care is a crucial part of your overall health. It is necessary for monitoring and managing your health conditions as well as preventing cardiovascular disease. Self-care includes the basics of healthy living and other things, such as adhering to a drug regimen and paying attention to new or worsening symptoms. It is estimated that self-care contributes to 40% of your health. Therefore, it is vital to always work with your healthcare providers so that any condition is properly diagnosed and managed.

LISTEN TO YOUR BODY

The rate of heart attacks and death due to untreated obstructive sleep apnea is becoming so alarming and heart breaking. It is important to check your blood pressure and sugar levels regularly. A lot of individuals are at risk because of their busy schedules, and they forget to take care of their health. Please remember to check your blood pressure regularly and know your numbers. Always check with your physician if you feel different in any way than you normally do, especially if you are always on the go. Your health is important, and your loved ones need you!

Walking is one of the great ways to maintain or improve your overall health. Walking for 30 minutes daily can improve heart health, reduce body fat, and strengthen the bones. It is one of the ways to be consistent in your exercise regimen.

If you have been inconsistent or have not been exercising at all, start with walking for at least 15 minutes a day and then increase to 30 minutes.

HEALTHY EATING ON THE GO

One of the biggest struggles most people face is unhealthy eating due to their very busy schedules. Quick and convenient foods are replaced by healthy, nourishing foods when we are on the go all the time. It is possible to eat healthily no matter how busy you are. Here is a list of healthy snack ideas to help when you get started: baby carrots and cucumber slices, grapes, nuts and raisins, sandwiches, hard-boiled eggs, and sliced or whole apples with nut butter.

When on a business trip or vacation, choose fresh, instead of processed food at the airport, and choose healthier food options at restaurants. Always drink lots of water to stay hydrated and avoid excessive intake of sugar. If you have a sweet tooth, you can look for naturally sweet products like fruits or yogurt. Non-perishable foods such as pretzels, trail mixes, protein or energy bars, and nuts that can satisfy hunger can be packed along during your trips or vacations. Remember to have a healthy breakfast; not having one makes you starve during the day, and this can make you look for unhealthy foods to eat.

Though you cannot pack liquids in your carry-on bag, there are some healthy options you can take with you. Wrapped whole food snack bars are a very good option, so you don't have to eat unhealthy food and snacks. You can use some apps such as 'find me gluten-free' for gluten-free restaurants or "Healthy Out" to keep your nutrition on track when eating out.

In summary, as a busy individual, schedule routine visits to your doctor for blood cholesterol and pressure screenings. Do not skip your annual wellness check; remember that awareness is key to early detection and prevention. Eat a well-balanced meal that includes fruits and vegetables, whole grains and lean proteins. Have a daily exercise routine; this can be as little as 5-10 minutes of walking during your lunch breaks.

Have a support system, surround yourself with loved ones who encourage you. Share your health goals with them; they can help and keep you accountable.

Daily checklist to improve your heart health:

- A heart-healthy meal
- Exercise daily
- Maintain a healthy weight
- No overeating
- Avoid smoking.
- Avoid alcohol

RECIPES

The following are some recipes that can help you on a healthy eating journey to improve your heart health. Meal plan 1 is designed to help the busy individual (always on the go and career individuals). Meal plan 2 and 3 can be used if you prefer some Nigerian or African meals. However, the meal plan is provided as a guide for you to know what type of meal you can eat and how to pair the food groups to your advantage.

- Pineapple Smoothie
- 1 cup spinach
- 1 cup water
- ½ cup pineapple frozen
- ½ cup mango frozen (optional)
- 1 banana
- 1 serving protein powder (optional)

Instructions

Add spinach to the blender with water. Blend together until all chunks are gone, well blended, and look like green water. Add other ingredients and blend well. Serve immediately or refrigerate until ready to drink.

Blueberry Banana Smoothie

- ½ cup spinach
- 1 cup almond milk
- ½ cup blueberries
- ½ cup strawberries
- 1 banana
- 1 serving protein powder (optional)

Instructions:

Add spinach and milk and blend until smooth.

Add fruits and blend.

Serve immediately or refrigerate until ready to drink.

Blueberry Kale Smoothie

- ½ cup spinach
- 1 cup almond milk (optional)
- ½ cup blueberries
- ½ cup kale
- 1 serving protein powder (optional)

Instructions:

Add spinach and milk, blend until smooth.

Add fruits and blend.

Serve immediately or refrigerate until ready to drink.

Berry Kale Smoothie

- ½ cup spinach
- 1 cup almond milk (optional) or water
- ½ cup blueberries
- ½ cup strawberries
- ½ cup kale
- 1 serving protein powder (optional)

Instructions:

Add spinach and milk, blend until smooth.

Add fruits, water, and blend.

Serve immediately or refrigerate until ready to drink.

Strawberry Banana Smoothie

- 1 cup strawberries frozen
- 1 banana
- 1 cup almond milk
- 1 cup ice or water
- 1 tbsp chia seeds (optional)
- 1 serving protein powder (optional)

Instructions:

Blend all ingredients until smooth.

Serve immediately or refrigerate until ready to drink.

Apple Kale Smoothie

- 1 cup fresh kale/ spinach
- 1 cup water
- 1 green apple cored

Instructions:

Blend all ingredients until smooth.

Serve immediately or refrigerate until ready to drink.

Chicken cabbage wrap

Remove any excess fat or skin from the chicken breast and discard. Cut the chicken into small pieces.

Place the cut chicken into a large bowl with the salt, pepper, onions, and mix. You can grill or air fry the chicken. Add all the chicken back into the wok or pan; add some green onions (optional) and a tablespoon of olive or vegetable oil. Add some red pepper flakes if you like, stir while cooking till the green onions are soft (2-3 minutes). Remove from heat, serve in cabbage leaves, and enjoy.

Basic Avocado toast sandwich

- 1 slice whole grain-toast
- 1/2 avocado sliced or mashed
- salt and pepper to taste
- red pepper flakes to taste

Remove half an avocado from its shell and pit and place it in a small bowl. Lightly mash it with a fork and add salt and pepper, or slice it.

Spread the avocado mixture over the toast and top with red pepper flakes.

For Avocado Toast with Egg

- 1 egg cooked the way you like it
- 5 cherry tomatoes sliced (optional)
- salt and pepper to taste

Remove half an avocado from its shell. Lightly mash it with salt and pepper or slice it.

Spread the avocado over the toast and top with sliced cherry tomatoes, egg, salt, and pepper. Slice the boiled egg and add to it.

Spicy broccoli corn sauté with salmon

- 1 cup broccoli florets
- 1 cup frozen sweet. corn
- 1 salmon

Pour the broccoli florets and sweet corn into a pot; add onion, pepper flakes, and salt to taste, and season. Cook on low heat for about 5-10 mins (till the broccoli is soft and cooked). Serve with grilled salmon.

Salad dressing: use your choice of salad dressing. Vinaigrette, Avocado or Ranch, but not more than 1 tablespoon.

Salmon and caesar salad

- 1 cup caesar salad
- 1 tablespoon dressing.
- Add salad dressing to the salad and mix thoroughly. Serve it with grilled or pan-seared salmon.

Egg salad sandwich

- 1 cup caesar salad
- 1 tablespoon dressing.
- 1 boiled egg

Add salad dressing to the salad and mix thoroughly. Slice the boiled egg and mix in the salad. Serve with 2-4 slices of whole wheat or whole grain bread (as a sandwich).

Quick vegetable sauté with rice

- 3 cups of spinach (or vegetable of choice)
- 1 red bell pepper
- 1 habanero (optional)
- 1 medium-sized onion
- 1 tablespoon of oil (olive, vegetable or palm oil)
- 2 cups frozen spinach (vegetable of choice)
- salt to taste

Pour the frozen spinach into the pot or saucepan, and add the chopped red bell pepper, onions, and habanero (optional). Stir and allow to cook for about 2-3 minutes. Add the vegetable oil (if using palm oil, add it after it has been heated for about 1 minute), and salt or seasoning to taste. Remember to use seasonings sparingly. Stir the vegetables and allow to cook for some time using low or medium heat. Serve it with 1 cup of cooked rice and your choice of grilled protein (fish or chicken). You should get 2-3 servings from the sautéed vegetable.

Vegetable fried rice and chicken

- 2 cups of rice
- 4 cups of chicken broth
- 1 cup (fresh) mixed bell peppers
- 1 cup of chopped onions and garlic
- 2 cups of frozen mixed vegetables
- 1 – 2 teaspoons of seasoning powder
- 1/4 teaspoon of salt (if needed)
- 2 teaspoons of ground curry
- 2 tablespoons of olive oil

Wash all vegetables, cut and set aside.

Add broth to a clean pot; ratio of rice to broth is 1:2 (1 cup of rice, 2 cups of broth), and add the curry. Let the broth boil, and then add the washed rice and let it cook for about 20-25 minutes. Set the cooked rice aside, then begin frying the vegetables (red bell pepper, mixed vegetables). Season the vegetable with little salt, and any seasoning you like (not too much). Add the thawed shrimp and fry together for about three minutes. Add the already cooked rice and stir fry till your desired taste. Serve it with grilled chicken or salmon or choice of fish.

IMPORTANT THINGS TO NOTE WHEN COOKING YOUR MEALS:

1. Note that only 1 cup of cooked rice (jollof, white or brown rice, fried rice) at a meal is okay at meals. You can enjoy your meal with lots of vegetables and fish or chicken.
2. When making African or Nigerian swallow, cup of garri, fufu, etc, is a good portion to be served with lots of vegetables and fish or chicken. Limit red meat as much as possible.
3. When making scrambled eggs, 1 tablespoon of olive oil or vegetable oil is good for 1 egg, and 2 tablespoon for two eggs.
4. Limit the use of salt when cooking; add your spices first and add a little salt to taste.
5. Air fry, grill, or boil your proteins (fish, chicken, turkey). And limit frying them.

These recipes and meal plans are a guide to help you eat healthy and are not meant to replace instructions given by your health care providers.

Please note that the information provided in this eBook is not intended to replace consultation with a qualified medical professional. We encourage you to inform your physician of changes you make to your lifestyle and discuss these with him or her. For questions or concerns about any medical conditions you may have, please contact your doctor.

The information provided is not intended to diagnose, treat, cure or prevent any disease. If you are pregnant, nursing, taking medication, or have a medical condition, consult your physician before making any changes to your diet.

Notes Date........... /...........

Notes Date........... /...........

Notes Date............ /............

Notes Date............ /............

Notes Date............ /............

Notes Date............ /............

GROCERY SHOPPING LIST

A well-planned grocery list can save you time and money at the grocery store; helping you stick to your healthy eating plan.

You can organize your list using the different aisles.

Produce

- Fruit: oranges, bananas, apples, pineapples, mangoes, strawberries, blueberries etc.
- Vegetables: kale, sweet potatoes, pumpkin leaves (ugwu), Jute leaves (ewedu), baby spinach, broccoli, carrot sticks, etc.

Colorful fruits and vegetables are nutritious. Buy fruits and vegetables that are locally grown and in season to save money.

Meat and Seafood

- Skinless chicken or turkey breasts
- Ground turkey or chicken
- Salmon, mackerel, or your favorite seafood
- Reduced-sodium lunchmeat (turkey, roast beef)

If you buy red meat, choose lean beef, look for sirloins, tenderloin, top sirloin, round steaks and roasts such as top round, bottom round, round tip.

Eat ground chicken or ground turkey breast instead of ground beef. These are much lower in fat.

Bakery and Bread

On Your List:

- Whole wheat bread
- Whole-grain flour tortillas

Look for the words "whole wheat" or "whole wheat flour" as the first ingredient on the label.

Choose whole-grain breads that contain at least 3 to 4 grams of fiber and have less than 100 calories per slice.

Pasta and Rice

- Brown rice
- Whole wheat or whole-grain pasta

Note that whole grains are best if you need to make a choice.

Oils, Sauces, Salad Dressings, and Condiments

- Tomato sauce
- Salsa
- Extra virgin olive oil, olive oil, nonfat cooking spray, palm oil.
- Hot pepper sauce

Many sauces and condiments are very high in sodium and sugar. Look for low sodium and sugar-free varieties.

Cereals and Breakfast Foods

- Whole-grain or multigrain cereals
- Instant oatmeal
- Whole-grain cereal bars

Buy cereals and cereal bars that are high in fiber and low in sugar. Use berries, dried fruit, or nuts to add sweetness to your cereal.

Soups and Canned Goods

- Diced or whole peeled tomatoes
- Tuna or salmon packed in water
- Low-sodium soups and broths

Check the label to see how much sodium is in canned vegetables and soups. Look for lower-sodium options, low sodium is defined as 140mg or less per serving. Rinse the canned foods before cooking, about 40 percent of the sodium can be removed by rinsing in some cases.

When buying canned fruits, choose brands that are packed in juice instead of syrup.

Snacks and Crackers

- Whole-grain crackers
- Dried fruit: prunes, raisins, cranberries
- Nuts: almonds, peanuts, cashews, walnuts, pecans, pistachios (unsalted and roasted)
- Seeds: sunflower seeds, sesame seeds, whole or ground flaxseeds
- Peanut butter, almond, or soy butter
- Dark chocolate
- Snack bars

Drinks

- Unsweetened green and flavored teas
- Calcium-fortified orange juice
- Sparkling water

Juice should be 100% fruit juice.

Frozen Foods

- Frozen vegetables: broccoli, spinach, peas, and carrots (no sauce)
- Frozen fruit: strawberries, raspberries, blueberries (without added sugar)
- Frozen shrimp
- Pre-portioned, low-fat ice cream or frozen yogurt
- Whole-grain waffles
- Whole-grain vegetable pizza

Buy frozen vegetables and add to soups, stews and meals.

Low-fat frozen yogurt blended with frozen fruit makes a quick, healthy smoothie.

Dairy, Cheese, and Eggs

- Skim or low-fat milk or soymilk
- Fat-free or low-fat yogurt
- Fat-free or low-fat cottage cheese
- Low-fat cheese or string cheese snacks
- Eggs or egg substitutes
- Firm tofu
- Butter (with no hydrogenated oils)

Choose plain yogurt instead of flavored ones as they can be high in sugar and calories. A tablespoon of fresh fruit can add flavor to your plain yogurt.

Notes Date............ /............

Notes Date............ /............

Notes Date............ /............

Notes Date............ /............

Notes Date............ /............

Notes Date............ /............

HEARTYNFIT BLOOD PRESSURE LOG

NAME: ____ MONTH: ____________________________

DAY	TIME	SYSTOLIC (UPPER)	DIASTOLIC (LOWER)	HEART RATE	NOTES
1					
2					
3					
4					
5					
6					
7					
8					
9					
10					
11					
12					
13					
14					
15					
16					
17					
18					
19					
20					
21					
22					
23					
24					
25					
26					
27					
28					
29					
30					
31					

HEARTYNFIT BLOOD PRESSURE LOG

NAME: ____________________ MONTH: ____________________

DAY	TIME	SYSTOLIC (UPPER)	DIASTOLIC (LOWER)	HEART RATE	NOTES
1					
2					
3					
4					
5					
6					
7					
8					
9					
10					
11					
12					
13					
14					
15					
16					
17					
18					
19					
20					
21					
22					
23					
24					
25					
26					
27					
28					
29					
30					
31					

HEARTYNFIT BLOOD PRESSURE LOG

NAME: ______________________ MONTH: ______________________

DAY	TIME	SYSTOLIC (UPPER)	DIASTOLIC (LOWER)	HEART RATE	NOTES
1					
2					
3					
4					
5					
6					
7					
8					
9					
10					
11					
12					
13					
14					
15					
16					
17					
18					
19					
20					
21					
22					
23					
24					
25					
26					
27					
28					
29					
30					
31					

HEALTHY HABIT TRACKER

	M	T	W	T	F	S	S
WATER	○	○	○	○	○	○	○
EXERCISE FOR 30 MINS	○	○	○	○	○	○	○
NO SODA	○	○	○	○	○	○	○
JOURNALING	○	○	○	○	○	○	○
HEALTHY EATING	○	○	○	○	○	○	○
SLEEP	○	○	○	○	○	○	○

TO DO LIST

-
-
-
-
-
-
-
-
-

NOTES

-
-
-
-
-
-
-
-
-

HEALTHY HABIT TRACKER

	M	T	W	T	F	S	S
WATER	○	○	○	○	○	○	○
EXERCISE FOR 30 MINS	○	○	○	○	○	○	○
NO SODA	○	○	○	○	○	○	○
JOURNALING	○	○	○	○	○	○	○
HEALTHY EATING	○	○	○	○	○	○	○
SLEEP	○	○	○	○	○	○	○

TO DO LIST

NOTES

HEALTHY HABIT TRACKER

	M	T	W	T	F	S	S
WATER	○	○	○	○	○	○	○
EXERCISE FOR 30 MINS	○	○	○	○	○	○	○
NO SODA	○	○	○	○	○	○	○
JOURNALING	○	○	○	○	○	○	○
HEALTHY EATING	○	○	○	○	○	○	○
SLEEP	○	○	○	○	○	○	○

TO DO LIST

-
-
-
-
-
-
-
-
-

NOTES

-
-
-
-
-
-
-
-
-

HEALTHY HABIT TRACKER

	M	T	W	T	F	S	S
WATER	○	○	○	○	○	○	○
EXERCISE FOR 30 MINS	○	○	○	○	○	○	○
NO SODA	○	○	○	○	○	○	○
JOURNALING	○	○	○	○	○	○	○
HEALTHY EATING	○	○	○	○	○	○	○
SLEEP	○	○	○	○	○	○	○

TO DO LIST

NOTES

HEALTHY HABIT TRACKER

	M	T	W	T	F	S	S
WATER	○	○	○	○	○	○	○
EXERCISE FOR 30 MINS	○	○	○	○	○	○	○
NO SODA	○	○	○	○	○	○	○
JOURNALING	○	○	○	○	○	○	○
HEALTHY EATING	○	○	○	○	○	○	○
SLEEP	○	○	○	○	○	○	○

TO DO LIST

- ....
- ....
- ....
- ....
- ....
- ....
- ....
- ....
- ....

NOTES

- ....
- ....
- ....
- ....
- ....
- ....
- ....
- ....
- ....

HEALTHY HABIT TRACKER

	M	T	W	T	F	S	S
WATER	○	○	○	○	○	○	○
EXERCISE FOR 30 MINS	○	○	○	○	○	○	○
NO SODA	○	○	○	○	○	○	○
JOURNALING	○	○	○	○	○	○	○
HEALTHY EATING	○	○	○	○	○	○	○
SLEEP	○	○	○	○	○	○	○

TO DO LIST

-
-
-
-
-
-
-
-
-

NOTES

-
-
-
-
-
-
-
-
-

HEALTHY HABIT TRACKER

	M	T	W	T	F	S	S
WATER	○	○	○	○	○	○	○
EXERCISE FOR 30 MINS	○	○	○	○	○	○	○
NO SODA	○	○	○	○	○	○	○
JOURNALING	○	○	○	○	○	○	○
HEALTHY EATING	○	○	○	○	○	○	○
SLEEP	○	○	○	○	○	○	○

TO DO LIST

-
-
-
-
-
-
-
-
-

NOTES

-
-
-
-
-
-
-
-
-

HEALTHY HABIT TRACKER

	M	T	W	T	F	S	S
WATER	○	○	○	○	○	○	○
EXERCISE FOR 30 MINS	○	○	○	○	○	○	○
NO SODA	○	○	○	○	○	○	○
JOURNALING	○	○	○	○	○	○	○
HEALTHY EATING	○	○	○	○	○	○	○
SLEEP	○	○	○	○	○	○	○

TO DO LIST

-
-
-
-
-
-
-
-
-

NOTES

-
-
-
-
-
-
-
-
-

HEALTHY HABIT TRACKER

	M	T	W	T	F	S	S
WATER	○	○	○	○	○	○	○
EXERCISE FOR 30 MINS	○	○	○	○	○	○	○
NO SODA	○	○	○	○	○	○	○
JOURNALING	○	○	○	○	○	○	○
HEALTHY EATING	○	○	○	○	○	○	○
SLEEP	○	○	○	○	○	○	○

TO DO LIST

-
-
-
-
-
-
-
-
-

NOTES

-
-
-
-
-
-
-
-
-

HEALTHY HABIT TRACKER

	M	T	W	T	F	S	S
WATER	○	○	○	○	○	○	○
EXERCISE FOR 30 MINS	○	○	○	○	○	○	○
NO SODA	○	○	○	○	○	○	○
JOURNALING	○	○	○	○	○	○	○
HEALTHY EATING	○	○	○	○	○	○	○
SLEEP	○	○	○	○	○	○	○

TO DO LIST

-
-
-
-
-
-
-
-
-

NOTES

-
-
-
-
-
-
-
-
-

HEALTHY HABIT TRACKER

	M	T	W	T	F	S	S
WATER	○	○	○	○	○	○	○
EXERCISE FOR 30 MINS	○	○	○	○	○	○	○
NO SODA	○	○	○	○	○	○	○
JOURNALING	○	○	○	○	○	○	○
HEALTHY EATING	○	○	○	○	○	○	○
SLEEP	○	○	○	○	○	○	○

TO DO LIST

-
-
-
-
-
-
-
-
-

NOTES

-
-
-
-
-
-
-
-
-

HEALTHY HABIT TRACKER

	M	T	W	T	F	S	S
WATER	○	○	○	○	○	○	○
EXERCISE FOR 30 MINS	○	○	○	○	○	○	○
NO SODA	○	○	○	○	○	○	○
JOURNALING	○	○	○	○	○	○	○
HEALTHY EATING	○	○	○	○	○	○	○
SLEEP	○	○	○	○	○	○	○

TO DO LIST

-
-
-
-
-
-
-
-
-

NOTES

-
-
-
-
-
-
-
-
-

weekly Meal Plan 1

MONDAY

Breakfast	Lunch	Dinner	Snack+ exercise
strawberry banana smoothie	egg salad sandwich	salmon ceasar salad	1 cup low-fat greek yogurt 30 mins walk

TUESDAY

Breakfast	Lunch	Dinner	Snack & exercise
blueberry kale smoothie	vegetable fried rice and chicken	sauteed spinach and fish	1 oz unsalted nuts 1 med cucumber 30 mins walk

WEDNESDAY

Breakfast	Lunch	Dinner	Snack & exercise
Strawberry banana smoothie	Avocado toast sandwich	chicken and vegetable salad with rice	1 cup low-fat greek yogurt 30 mins walk.

THURSAY

Breakfast	Lunch	Dinner	Snack & exercise
apple kale smoothie	chicken cabbage wrap	tilapia with vegetable sauce	1 fruit e.g.apple 30 mins walk

FRIDAY

Breakfast	Lunch	Dinner	Snack & exercise
pineapple smoothie	egg salad sandwich	quick vegetable saute with rice	1 cup low-fat greek yogurt 30 mins walk

SATURDAY

Breakfast	Lunch	Dinner	Snack & exercise
strawberry banana smoothie	chicken cabbage wrap	tilapia/croaker with vegetable sauce	1 oz unsalted nuts 1 medium banana 30 mins walk

SUNDAY

Breakfast	Lunch	Dinner	Snack & exercise
blue berry banana smoothie	Avocado toast sandwich	Vegetable fried rice and chicken	1 serving of fruit e.g berries. 30 mins walk

weekly Meal Plan 2

Day	Breakfast	Lunch	Dinner	Snacks + exercise
MONDAY	3 medium slicess Yam and egg	1 cup cooked rice and beans with fish or chicken	tilapia with vegtable sauce	1oz unsalted nuts 1 medium banana. 30 mins walk
TUESDAY	Apple kale smoothie	1/3 cup swallow, vegetables and fish	chicken and vegetable salad with rice	1 cup low-fat greek yogurt 30 mins walk
WEDNESDAY	1 cup cooked oat with moinoin	1 cup cooked jollof rice, tilapia with vegetable sauce	salmon ceasar salad	1 oz unsalted nuts 1 medium banana. 30 mins walk
THURSAY	Wheat bread and egg	1/3 cup swallow, okro soup and fish	chicken and vegetable salad with rice	1 serving of fruit e.g berries. 30 mins walk
FRIDAY	1 cup cooked oat and moinmoin	1 cup cooked rice tilapia with vegetable sauce	salmon ceasar salad	1 cup low-fat greek yogurt 30 mins walk
SATURDAY	Avocado toast sandwich	chicken cabbage wrap	1 medium boiled plantain, vegetable and fish	1 oz unsalted nut 1 cucumber 30 mins walk
SUNDAY	blue berry banana smoothie	1/3 cup swallow, vegetables and fish	Vegetable fried rice and chicken	1 serv. of fruit e.g apple. 30 mins walk

weekly Meal Plan 3

MONDAY

Breakfast	Lunch	Dinner	Snacks + exercise
Avocado toast sandwich	1 cup cooked rice and beans with fish or chicken	Fish/vegetable sauce, 1 boiled unripe plantain	1oz unsalted nuts 1 medium banana 30 mins walk

TUESDAY

Breakfast	Lunch	Dinner	Snacks + exercise
Apple kale smoothie	1/3 cup swallow, vegetables and fish	chicken and vegetable sauce with rice	1 cup low-fat greek yogurt 30 mins walk

WEDNESDAY

Breakfast	Lunch	Dinner	Snacks + exercise
1 cup cooked oat with moinoin	tilapia with vegetable sauce	salmon ceasar salad/cole slaw & 1 med. chicken breast	1 oz unsalted nuts 1 medium banana 30 mins walk

THURSAY

Breakfast	Lunch	Dinner	Snacks +exercise
Wheat bread and scrambled egg	1/3 cup swallow, okro soup and fish	Beans and plantain with fish (optional)	1 serv. of fruit e.g berries. 30 mins walk

FRIDAY

Breakfast	Lunch	Dinner	Snacks + exercise
1 cup cooked oat and moinmoin	1 cup cooked rice tilapia with vegetable sauce	salmon ceasar salad	1 cup low-fat greek yogurt 30 mins walk

SATURDAY

Breakfast	Lunch	Dinner	Snacks + exercise
strawberry banana smoothie	chicken cabbage wrap	1 medium boiled plantain, vegetable and fish	1 oz unsalted nuts a cucumber 30 mins walk

SUNDAY

Breakfast	Lunch	Dinner	Snacks + exercise
Apple kale smoothie	1/3 cup swallow, vegetables and fish	Vegetable fried rice and chicken	1 serving of fruit e.g berries, apple. 30 mins walk

weekly Meal Plan 4

MONDAY

Breakfast	Lunch	Dinner	Snack+ exercise
strawberry banana smoothie	egg salad sandwich	salmon ceasar salad	1 cup low-fat greek yogurt 30 mins walk

TUESDAY

Breakfast	Lunch	Dinner	Snack & exercise
blueberry kale smoothie	vegetable fried rice and chicken	sauteed spinach and fish	1 oz unsalted nuts 1 med cucumber 30 mins walk

WEDNESDAY

Breakfast	Lunch	Dinner	Snack & exercise
Strawberry banana smoothie	Avocado toast sandwich	chicken and vegetable salad with rice	1 cup low-fat greek yogurt 30 mins walk

THURSAY

Breakfast	Lunch	Dinner	Snack & exercise
apple kale smoothie	chicken cabbage wrap	tilapia with vegetable sauce	1 fruit (e.g.apple)30 mins walk

FRIDAY

Breakfast	Lunch	Dinner	Snack & exercise
pineapple smoothie	egg salad sandwich	quick vegetable saute with rice	1 cup low-fat greek yogurt 30 mins walk

SATURDAY

Breakfast	Lunch	Dinner	Snack & exercise
strawberry banana smoothie	chicken cabbage wrap	tilapia/croaker with vegetable sauce	1 oz unsalted nuts, 1 medium banana. 30 mins walk

SUNDAY

Breakfast	Lunch	Dinner	Snack & exercise
blue berry banana smoothie	Avocado toast sandwich	Vegetable fried rice and chicken	1 serv. of fruit e.g apple 30 mins walk

ABOUT AUTHOR

Dr. Fisayo is a seasoned health and wellness professional with expertise in program development and implementation, specializing in nutrition education, counseling, health promotion, global and public health.

Certified as a Health Coach, Dr. Fisayo holds specializations as a Fitness Nutrition Specialist, Behavior Change Specialist, and Weight Management Specialist by the American Council on Exercise (ACE).

She is the Founder and Lead Wellness Consultant at HeartyNFit in Katy, Texas, she is dedicated to empowering individuals to overcome health challenges through proactive coaching, addressing high blood cholesterol, blood pressure, stress, and weight management.

Employing motivational interviewing and SMART goal setting, she guides clients toward sustainable behavior change.

Dr, Fisayo's diverse background, certifications, and contributions in the health and wellness domain position her as an asset in corporate wellness programs and health-focused initiatives. Her commitment to global and public health, particularly in chronic disease prevention and management, underscores her passion to create a positive impact on individuals and communities worldwide.

Connect with her on social media:

Facebook: HeartyNFit
Instagram: @heartynfit
LinkedIn: Fisayo Adegoke, DHSc.

Notes Date............ /............

Notes Date............ /............

Notes Date........... /...........

Notes Date........... /...........

Notes Date............ /............

Notes Date............ /............

Notes

Date........... /...........

Notes

Date........... /...........

Notes Date........... /...........

Notes Date........... /...........

Notes Date............ /............

Notes Date............ /............

Notes Date............ /............

....

....

....

....

....

....

....

....

....

....

....

....

Notes Date............ /............

....

....

....

....

....

....

....

....

....

....

....

....

Notes Date........... /...........

Notes Date........... /...........

Notes Date........... /...........

....

....

....

....

....

....

....

....

....

....

....

....

Notes Date........... /...........

....

....

....

....

....

....

....

....

....

....

....

....

Notes Date.............. /..............

Notes Date.............. /..............

REFERENCES

American Heart Association. "My cholesterol guide". Assessed October 30, 2023. My Cholesterol Guide: Taken Action. Live Healthy! (heart.org)

American Heart Association. "What is cholesterol." Assessed October 29, 2023. What is Cholesterol? | American Heart Association

American Heart Association. "Understanding Blood Pressure Readings". Assessed November 14, 2023. Understanding Blood Pressure Readings | American Heart Association

British Heart Foundation (June 2023). Global Heart and Circulatory Diseases Fact Sheet. www.bhf.org.uk

Heart disease (March 15, 2023). www.cdc.gov

Signs and symptoms of heart disease in men (medicalnewstoday.com)

Health Direct. "Cholesterol." www.healthdirect.gov.au/cholesterol#types

Cholesterol – what to do if your cholesterol is too high | healthdirect

Healthline. "Is Goat Meat Healthy? All You Need to Know." Goat Meat: Nutrients, Benefits, Downsides & More (healthline.com)

Center for Disease Control and Prevention. (June 3, 2022). Healthy Weight, Nutrition and Physical Activity. About Adult BMI | Healthy Weight, Nutrition, and Physical Activity | CDC
InformedHealth.org [Internet]. Cologne, Germany: Institute for Quality and Efficiency in Health Care (IQWiG); 2006-. High cholesterol: Overview. 2013 Aug 14 [Updated 2017 Sep 7]. Available from: https://www.ncbi.nlm.nih.

gov/books/NBK279318/

John Hopkins Medicine. "Lipid Panel."Assessed October 30, 2023. www.johnhopkinsmedicine.org/health/treatment/tests-and-therapies/lipid-panel

Lipid Panel | Johns Hopkins Medicine

Lee SH, Moore LV, Park S, Harris DM, Blanck HM. Adults Meeting Fruit and Vegetable Intake Recommendations — United States, 2019. MMWR Morb Mortal Wkly Rep 2022;71:1–9. DOI: http://dx.doi.org/10.15585/mmwr.mm7101a1

Mayo Clinic. "Heart attack. "Assessed, October 30, 2023. Heart attack - Symptoms & causes - Mayo Clinic

National Heart, Blood and Lung Institute. "How the heart works." Assessed October 29, 2023. How the Heart Works - The Heart | NHLBI, NIH

Pem, D., & Jeewon, R. (2015). Fruit and Vegetable Intake: Benefits and Progress of Nutrition Education Interventions- Narrative Review Article. Iranian journal of public health, 44(10), 1309–1321.

Prairie View A & M. " Goat meat, a health choice". Assessed November, 4, 2023. goatmeat_approved.pdf (pvamu.edu)

Rêgo, M. L., Cabral, D. A., Costa, E. C., & Fontes, E. B. (2019). Physical Exercise for Individuals with Hypertension: It Is Time to Emphasize its Benefits on the Brain and Cognition. Clinical Medicine Insights. Cardiology, 13, 1179546819839411. https://doi.org/10.1177/1179546819839411

Made in the USA
Las Vegas, NV
03 November 2026

57424295R00062